Keto Diet Recipes for Women Over 50

Over 50

50 Simply and Tasty Recipes for Your Sweet Moments of Relax

Rose Pope

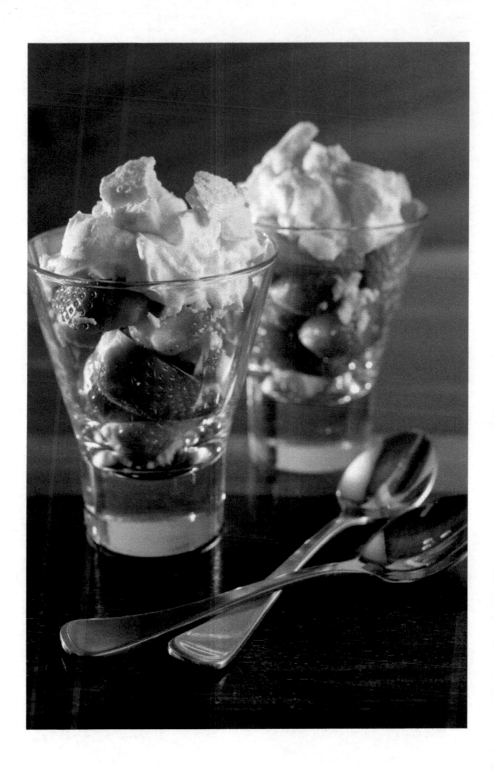

sources. Please consult a licensed professional before attempting any techniques outlined in this book.

By reading this document, the reader agrees that under no circumstances is the author responsible for any losses, direct or indirect, which are incurred as a result of the use of information contained within this document, including, but not limited to, — errors, omissions, or inaccuracies.

Table of Contents

Desserts Recipes

1 Low Carb Sugar-Free Peppermint Patties

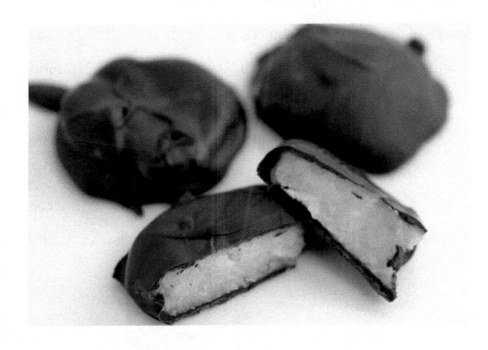

Servings: 24 | **Time:** 30 mins | **Difficulty:** Easy

Nutrients per serving: Calories: 90 kcal | Fat: 1g | Carbohydrates: 61g | Protein: 0g | Fiber: 2g

Ingredients

1/4 Tsp. peppermint extract

1/2 cup heavy cream (or dairy-free alternative)

6 1/2 cup powdered erythritol (like powdered swerve)

2 cups low carb chocolate chips

Method

1. Using parchment paper to prepare the large baking sheets.

2. Put 1 Tbsp. of milk, peppermint oil, and powdered erythritol in a large mixing bowl. Add the remaining 1 Tbsp. of cream one at a time, slowly. Continue to blend until it starts shaping a ball.

3. Pick one tbsp of the dough you have made, roll it into a small ball, and press it flat. And continue until all the patties of peppermint are made. Freeze yourself for 1 hour.

4. Add chocolate chips and microwave for 30 seconds in a microwave-safe cup, mix, and proceed until the chocolate fully melts. (1.5 minutes approx)

5. Dip the peppermint patties into molten chocolate easily with a fork, tap on the bowl edge to extract excess chocolate, and

put back on parchment paper to make the placement of chocolate.

6.   If you want to speed up the chocolate sets, put 5-10 minutes in the freezer.

7.   Store in an airtight jar.

2   Crustless Pumpkin Pie

Servings: 9 | **Time:** 1 hr 8 mins | **Difficulty:** Easy

Nutrients per serving: Calories: 40 kcal | Fat: 1g | Carbohydrates: 23g | Protein: 2g | Fiber: 2g

Ingredients

2 large eggs

1/4 Tsp. salt

1/2 cup erythritol

1 Tsp. pure liquid stevia (optional)

1 Tsp. ground cinnamon

1 Tbsp. pumpkin spice

1 cup unsweetened almond milk (or heavy cream)

1 (15 oz) can of pure pumpkin puree

Method

1.   Preheat the oven to 425°F

2.   In a mixing cup, whisk together all the ingredients.

3.   If you would like, spill it into an oiled 8x8 plate or pie pan.

4.   Then raise the heat to 350 °F—Bake for 15 minutes. For a further 35-40 minutes, continue to bake, or until the pie is set up and cooked. The knife in the middle should come out clean.

3   Low Carb Chocolate Covered Bacon

Servings: 12 | **Time:** 25 mins | **Difficulty:** Easy

Nutrients per serving: Calories: 164 kcal | Fat: 16g | Carbohydrates: 6g | Protein: 2g | Fiber: 0g

Ingredients

1 cup low carb chocolate

12 wooden skewers

14 strips cooked bacon

Method

1.   Take bacon that is freshly hot and fried. Skewer through a piece of bacon carefully. Leave the bacon to cool perfectly.

2.   Create a baking sheet out of parchment paper.

3.   Add the low carb chocolate and microwave for about 30 seconds, swirl and repeat until the chocolate is fully melted in the microwaveable glass cup.

4　Low Carb Zucchini Bread

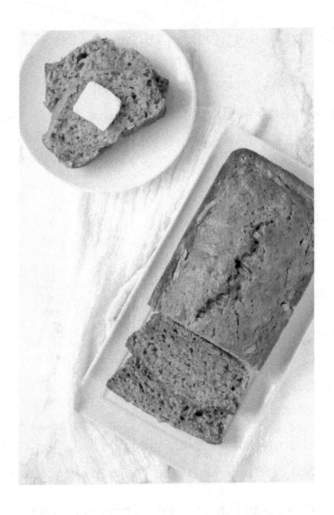

Servings: 18 | **Time**: 1 hr 10 mins | **Difficulty**: Easy

Nutrients per serving: Calories: 155 kcal | Fat: 15g | Carbohydrates: 9g | Protein: 5g | Fiber: 2g

Ingredients

1/2 cup monk fruit sweetener (+ 1/4 cup for more sweetness)

1/4 tsp. ground nutmeg

1/4 tsp. salt

1 1/2 cups almond flour

1/2 cup pecan pieces

1/2 cup coconut oil

1/2 tsp. pure liquid stevia

1 tbsp. baking powder

2 tsp. ground cinnamon

6 large eggs

1 tbsp. lemon zest

1 cup grated zucchini

Method

1. Preheat the oven to 350 °F.

2. In a medium to big mixing cup, combine all the ingredients.

3. Line parchment paper with a regular loaf pan and pour a batter into a pan.

4.   Bake for around 50-60 minutes, or until the knife inserted in the center is clean.

5.   Until slicing, cool fully.

5   Low Carb Chocolate Bars

Servings: 9 | **Time:** 10 mins | **Difficulty**: Easy

Nutrients per serving: Calories: 169 kcal | Fat: 18g | Carbohydrates: 8g | Protein: 0g | Fiber: 1g

Ingredients

10 drops pure liquid stevia

1 tsp. pure vanilla extract

1/2 cup unsweetened cocoa powder

1/4 cup erythritol

3/4 cup coconut oil, melted and hot

Method

1.   Using a safe microwave cup to heat the oil in the pot on the burner or in a microwave.

2.   Stir the remainder of the ingredients. When the oil is heated, then whisk to remove the lumps from a cocoa powder. It

will take a couple of minutes. When all is properly mixed, the mixture should be smooth and fluffy.

3.   Pour chocolate into a baking dish or chocolate mold or option lined with parchment and put in   a refrigerator for 2 hours or until the chocolate is completely hardened.

4.   Set the dish out for about 20-30 minutes on a counter to leave the chocolate melt a little before cutting.

5.   Keep in the refrigerator or freezer in an air-tight jar.

6   Low Carb Orange Almond Cake Bars

Servings: 28 | **Time:** 40 mins | **Difficulty:** Easy

Nutrients per serving: Calories: 84 kcal | Fat: 7g | Carbohydrates: 3g | Protein: 2g | Fiber: 1g

Ingredients

1 tsp. pure liquid stevia

4 large eggs

2 tsp. baking powder

1/2 cup unsalted butter (softened - I used a non-dairy butter) 1/2 cup coconut flour

1/2 tsp. orange extract

1/2 tsp. almond extract

1 1/4 cup fine-ground almond flour

1/8 tsp. salt

3/4 cup xylitol

1/4 cup powdered xylitol I just powdered my own in a spice grinder)

1/4 tsp. almond extract

1/4 cup sliced almonds

1 tsp. orange extract

1 tbsp. milk (you can use unsweetened almond milk)

Method

1.   Preheat the oven to 325 °F.

2.   Put parchment in it without oiling the pan and set aside using a quarter-size baking sheet.

3.   Whip the butter in a blender until smooth, then add the sweetener. Half the flour is added. Until this is introduced into the butter, all other ingredients continue to be added.

4.   It will have the consistency of whipped cream cheese or a whipped butter when the batter is finished. Thick, still tender. Scrap the dough onto the cookie sheet and spread the dough out uniformly over a cookie sheet to around 1/2 inch thickness using a recessed spatula.

5.   For 20 minutes, roast them. You can prepare the topping as it bakes. Whisk together the extracts, powdered sweetener, and about 2 tbsp in a small dish. For whatever milk you want to use.

6.   Move a bar dough to the cutting board when the bars are finished baking and allow it to cool completely. Place it in the freezer for a minimum of 2 hours.

7.   11. Mix the topping ingredients, except for the almonds. leave it to stay in the almond milk for around 5-10 min to reach the sweetener to dissolve completely.

8.   Scatter the icing over the bars with a spoon, and then finish with almonds. Split the dough   into thin strips. Use low carb hot chocolate to serve. Keep in a freezer until fit for serving. They are more like cookies and are better eaten with a fork.

7   Low Carb Coconut Vanilla Ice Cream

Servings: 4 | **Time:** 1 hr | **Difficulty:** Easy

Nutrients per serving: Calories: 411 kcal | Fat: 48g | Carbohydrates: 5g | Protein: 2g | Fiber: 3g

Ingredients

1/8 tsp. salt

1/4 cup erythritol

1/2 cup MCT oil

4 large egg yolks (pasteurized eggs are safest)

1 (15 oz.) can full-fat coconut milk

2 tsp. pure vanilla extract

Method

1.   In a blender, add all the ingredients, and mix for 20 seconds, or until all is well mixed.

2.   Move the blend to the ice cream maker and continue with the manual for the unit.

8   Keto Vanilla Cupcakes

Servings: 12 | **Time**: 30 mins | **Difficulty:** Easy

Nutrients per serving: Calories: 107 kcal | Fat: 10g | Carbohydrates: 8g | Protein: 3g | Fiber: 2g

Ingredients

3 Tbsp. unsalted butter, melted

2 whole eggs

1/4 Tsp. salt

1/4 cup powdered erythritol

1/4 cup brown sugar alternative

1/2 Tsp. vanilla extract

1/2 Tsp. baking soda

1/2 cup unsweetened almond milk

1 Tsp. baking powder

1 Tsp. apple cider vinegar

1 1/2 cups almond flour

Method

1. Preheat the oven to 350°F. Oiled or bake with cupcake liners to prepare a muffin tin.

2. Mix the almond milk and the vinegar in a small bowl and set aside.

3. Mix the dry products, almond flour, erythritol, baking powder, salt, baking soda, and brown sugar in a big cup.

4. Create a dry ingredient core and apply the mixture of eggs, butter, almond milk/vinegar, and vanilla extract. Mix once mixed properly.

5. Spoon the flour into the lined tin for baking. 3/4 complete filling of each tin. Bake for about 20-22 minutes, or until a toothpick comes out clean.

6. Leave them to cool completely before frosting and enjoy your favorite low carb frosting.

9 Low Carb Chocolate Ice Cream

Servings: 4 | **Time:** 1 hr | **Difficulty:** Easy

Nutrients per serving: Calories: 323 kcal | Fat: 34g | Carbohydrates: 16g | Protein: 4g | Fiber: 3g

Ingredients

4 large egg yolks (pasteurized are safest)

2 tsp. pure vanilla extract

2 cups unsweetened chocolate almond milk

10 drops pure liquid stevia

1/8 tsp. sea salt

1/4 cup powdered monk fruit

1/2 cup MCT oil

1 tbsp. unsweetened cocoa powder

Method

1.   In a blender, put all the ingredients and blend for 1 - 2 minutes.

2.   Put the mixture in your ice cream maker and operate as directed by the machine.

3.   Scoop and then enjoying

10 Keto Double Chocolate Cookie Dough

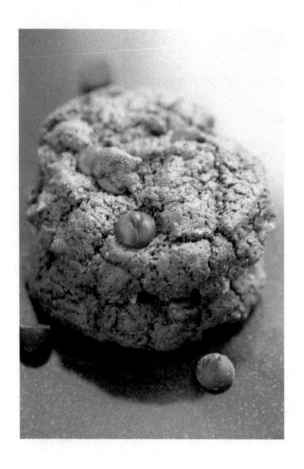

Servings: 32 | **Time:** 10 mins | **Difficulty:** Easy

Nutrients per serving: Calories: 58 kcal | Fat: 5g | Carbohydrates: 3g | Protein: 0g | Fiber: 1g

Ingredients

1/8 Tsp. liquid stevia

1/4 cup of low carb chocolate chips

1/2 cup softened butter

1/4 -1/2 cup of powdered erythritol

1/2 Tsp. sea salt

1/2 cup heavy cream or coconut milk for a dairy-free alternative
1/2 cup coconut flour

1 Tsp. vanilla extract

3 Tbsp. cocoa powder

Method

1.   Butter, vanilla extract, stevia, salt, erythritol, and the heavy cream are creamed together in a large bowl.

2.   Beat until well mixed with coconut flour and cocoa powder.

3.   Fold the chocolate chips together. Eat into bite-sized bits with a spoon or scoop as they become more stable after being stored in the fridge. Store it in the freezer.

11 Low Carb Keto Cream Cheese Frosting

Servings: 32 | **Time**: 10 mins | **Difficulty:** Easy

Nutrients per serving: Calories: 36 kcal | Fat: 3g | Carbohydrates: 9g | Protein: 0g

Ingredients

8 ounces cream cheese softened

2 cups powdered erythritol like powdered swerve

1/4 cup butter softened

Method

1.   Take a medium-sized mixing bowl, mix the cream cheese and butter slowly add the powdered sweetener until smooth with a hand mixer or a stand mixer.

2.   Onto your favorite low carbohydrates cupcakes or cake, pipe or ice and enjoy

12 Low Carb Raspberry Chocolate Sponge Cake

Servings: 12 | **Time:** 55 mins | **Difficulty:** Easy

Nutrients per serving: Calories: 195 kcal | Fat: 16g | Carbohydrates: 12g | Protein: 6g | Fiber: 5g

Ingredients

1/8 Tsp. pure liquid stevia

1/4 cup coconut flour

1/4 cup erythritol

1/4 cup melted butter or butter alternative

1 1/2 cups almond flour

1/2 Tsp. xanthan gum

1/2 cup whole milk or dairy-free alternative

1/2 cup raspberries

1/2 cup of low carb chocolate chips

1 Tsp. baking powder

1 Tsp. pure vanilla extract

4 large eggs

4 Tbsp. lemon juice

Method

1.   Preheat the oven to 350°F. Oiled with the cooking spray or oil to prepare a 9x13 pan.

2.   In a big dish, combine the almond flour, erythritol, xanthan gum, coconut flour, and baking powder.

3.   Build a well and apply extract, eggs, whole milk, liquid stevia, and lemon juice to the middle of dry ingredients. Mix before it is mixed properly.

4.   Fold in the raspberries and chocolate chips. Into a prepared pan, pour. Bake for about 35-40 minutes, or until the toothpick is clean.

13 Low Carb Dairy Free Raspberry Mousse

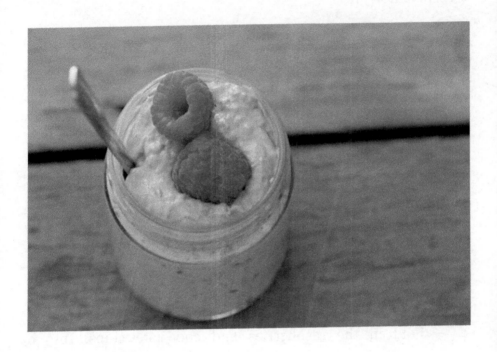

Servings: 4 | **Time:** 15 mins | **Difficulty:** Easy

Nutrients per serving: Calories: 201 kcal | Fat: 28g | Carbohydrates: 3.5g | Protein: 0.5g | Fiber: 2.5g

Ingredients

2 tbsp. erythritol or the low carb sweetener of your choice to taste

1 (4 oz.) package fresh raspberries

1 (15 oz.) can full-fat coconut milk (refrigerated for 2 days)

Method

1. Set aside a pair of raspberries for garnish while you are serving this to visitors.

2. In a blender, put all ingredients and blend until they become smooth.

3. Pour into the serving cups, then top and serve with a fresh raspberry.

14   Keto Low Carb Pumpkin Bars

Servings: 18 | **Time:** 2 hrs 15 mins | **Difficulty:** Easy

Nutrients per serving: Calories: 171 kcal | Fat: 13g | Carbohydrates: 14g | Protein: 2g | Fiber: 5g

Ingredients

1 (15 oz.) can full-fat coconut milk

1 (15 oz.) can pumpkin puree (not pumpkin pie filling)

1 tbsp. coconut flour

1 tsp. ground cinnamon

1 tsp. pure liquid stevia

1/2 cup erythritol or another low carb sweetener

16 oz. food-grade cocoa butter

2 tsp. pumpkin pie spice, no sugar added

Method

1.   Then melt the cocoa butter in a small-medium pot on low to medium heat.

2.   Stir in the milk from the coconut and then a pumpkin puree. To prevent burning, stir in all   the other ingredients and keep the heat on the low side. More of a custard consistency should thicken the mixture.

3.   Pour it into the parchment-lined casserole dish until it reaches that consistency, then put the dish for at least two hours in the freezer.

7.   Remove, cut, sprinkle with sliced pecan parts from the freezer, and enjoy.

8.   Store in a fridge the rest.

15   Low Carb Blackberry Ice Cream

Servings: 6 | **Time:** 25 mins | **Difficulty:** Easy

Nutrients per serving: Calories: 158 kcal | Fat: 14g | Carbohydrates: 31g | Protein: 2g | Fiber: 3g

Ingredients

1/4 tsp. almond extract (optional)

1/2 tsp. ground cinnamon

1/2 cup erythritol

1 (15 oz.) can full-fat coconut milk

1 tsp. pure vanilla extract

4 large whole egg yolks, set aside in a medium bowl

1 (6 oz.) package fresh blackberries

Method

1.   Bring coconut milk to a low boil in a medium cup.

2.   Stir in the cinnamon and the vanilla, and the cinnamon will break up any clumps.

3.   Take the heat-proof spoon or a small cup and gently pour about 1/4 of a cup of the hot milk into the eggs while whisking rapidly. Pour slowly and whisk immediately.

4.   When you've stirred the hot milk into the shell, gently pour the egg into a simmering pot of coconut oil. The egg temperature is steadily increased by this process so that it blends into the milk without making you scrambled eggs.

5.   Apply the erythritol to the pot of milk until you have the egg in it. With the potato masher or   a fork, add the blackberries and crush them.

6.   Remove that from the sun and cool in the refrigerator with all the batter.

7.   Shift to your ice cream maker until fully cooled and continue to the manufacturer's instructions for your computer. Store in a food-safe jar in the freezer until ready to taste.

16 Sugar-Free Marshmallows

Servings: 16 | **Time:** 1 day 30 mins | **Difficulty:** Easy

Nutrients per serving: Calories: 4 kcal | Fat: 1g | Carbohydrates: 14g | Protein: 1g

Ingredients

1 1/2 cups powdered erythritol (or favorite powdered sugar substitute)

1 cup of warm water

1/4 Tsp. sea salt

2 Tbsp. unflavored gelatin

2 Tsp. vanilla extract

Method

1.   In a wide dish, position 1/2 cup of the warm water. This dish should be big enough as the marshmallows in that bowl can be combined. You'll get a mess otherwise.

2.   Sprinkle gelatin on the top of hot water and whisk, set aside, before adding.

3.   Place the remaining half cup of water, powdered sugar replacement, and salt in a medium saucepan over medium-low heat. Whisk the components together until they are transparent. As soon as you see, bubbles start forming, extract them from the sun.

4.   In your large mixing cup, add the warm mixture into it. You have the little air in a mixture and shape stiff peaks using the hand mixer or a stand mixer with the whisk attachment, then whisk for about 15-20 minutes before the color changes from light brown to white.

5.   In an 8x8 baking dish, put the parchment paper. To help avoid sticking, dust with the powdered sweetener.

6.   In a lined baking dish, add the marshmallow mixture and refrigerate overnight. The dough on the surface can become solid and not soft.

7.   Use the parchment paper to clear it from the jar. Coat a bit of powdered sweetener with your sharp knife, carve it into the marshmallows, and make 16 squares. If the dough seems to be a little moist, you should sprinkle the marshmallows with a bit more erythritol to protect them from sticking. Store in an airtight jar.

17   Keto Coffee Popsicles

Servings: 4 | **Time:** 1 day | **Difficulty:** Easy

Nutrients per serving: Calories: 123 kcal | Fat: 14g | Carbohydrates: 0g | Protein: 0g | Fiber: 0g

Ingredients

stevia to taste (or maybe low carb sweetener you prefer)

4 tbsp. food-grade cocoa butter

1 tsp. pure vanilla extract

1 1/4 cup brewed coffee

Method

1.   Blend it all in a blender together.

2.   Pour and chill overnight in Popsicle molds.

18 Low Carb Sugar-Free Meringue Cookies

Servings: 24 | **Time:** 2 hrs 40 mins | **Difficulty:** Easy

Nutrients per serving: Calories: 2 kcal | Fat: 0g | Carbohydrates: 10g | Protein: 0g | Fiber: 0g

Ingredients

3 large egg whites at room temperature

1 Tsp. vanilla extract

1/2 cup erythritol

3/4 cup powdered erythritol

Method

1.   Preheat the oven to 200°F

2.   Line the baking sheet or oiled parchment paper with a non-stick silicone pad. The silicone mat fits best, I think.

3.   Add the egg whites to a medium bowl with a hand blender and beat for 1 minute at the medium- low level. Egg albumins should be frothy and white.

4.   Continue to blend at medium speed, add 1 tbsp of erythritol (powdered) at a time, and continue whisking until rigid peaks shape. The batter should be thick and shiny. Stir in the vanilla extract.

5.   On lined baking sheets, spoon meringue flour into mounds or spoon into the piping bag, then pipe into small mounds.

6.   Bake for 2.5 -3 hours or before the meringues on the outside is dried. And a parchment paper with the intact bottoms is discarded, and the centers inside are not sticky. Switch the oven off and inside the oven, allow them to cool.

7.   For up to 2 weeks, you can preserve it in an airtight container.

19   Keto Blackberry Clafoutis

Servings: 6 | **Time:** 50 mins | **Difficulty:** Easy

Nutrients per serving: Calories: 163 kcal | Fat: 13.4g | Carbohydrates: 7g | Protein: 3.7g | Fiber: 3.5g

Ingredients

Pinch of sea salt

2 Tbsp. plus

1 Tsp. butter

2 large eggs

2 cups blackberries

2 ½ Tbsp. coconut flour

½ Tsp. pure vanilla extract

½ Tsp. baking powder

⅓ cup powdered erythritol

⅓ cup heavy cream

¼ cup coconut milk, almond milk, OR cashew milk

Method

1.   Preheat the oven to 350 °F. Oiled up a 10" oval baking dish gently.

2.   At low pressure, heat a small saucepan. Melt the butter in a pan and then heat it until it becomes golden brown, take very good care, and not let it burn.

3.   Remove   the   container   from the   heating   and   stir   in   the   eggs, vanilla   extract, and erythritol Whiskey until the mixture becomes creamy and light in color.

4.   In the coconut flour, stir gently. Then add in the milk, yogurt, salt, and baking powder of the coconut. Mix until all the ingredients are well blended.

5.   Pour the mixture into the baking dish prepared and covered with blackberries—Bake in the middle for 40 minutes.

6.   The core will still be somewhat wobbly but will begin to set as it cools off. You can cook it for 5 - 10 minutes longer if you like a somewhat crispier clafoutis.

7.   Before eating, sprinkle with powdered erythritol, or finish with low carbohydrate vanilla ice cream or the whipped cream.

20 Pumpkin Spice Cupcakes With Marshmallow Frosting

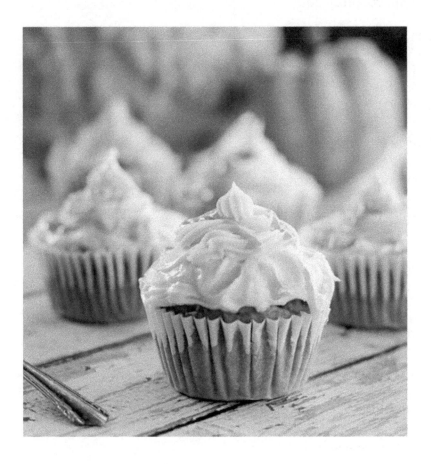

Servings: 6 | **Time:** 40 mins | **Difficulty**: Easy

Nutrients per serving: Calories: 2 kcal | Fat: 60g | Carbohydrates: 7g | Protein: 13g | Fiber: 7g

Ingredients

FOR THE PUMPKIN SPICE CUPCAKES:

3 Tbsp. coconut flour

2 Tbsp. chopped walnuts

2 Tbsp. coconut oil, butter, or butter flavored coconut oil (melted)

2 large eggs, separated

1 Tsp. pure vanilla extract

1 Tsp. baking powder

1 ½ Tsp. Pumpkin Pie Spice

¾ Tsp. ground chia seeds

¾ cup blanched almond flour

½ Tsp. apple cider vinegar

⅓ cup plus 1 Tbsp. pumpkin puree (unsweetened)

¼ Tsp. of sea salt

¼ cup almond milk (unsweetened)

¼ cup golden monk fruit

FOR THE MARSHMALLOW FROSTING:

¼ Tsp. cream of tartar

¼ Tsp. of sea salt

1 cup powdered erythritol or monk fruit

1 Tsp. pure vanilla extract

4 large egg white, room temperature

Method

FOR THE PUMPKIN SPICE CUPCAKES:

1.   Preheat the oven to 350°F.

2.   Mix the almond flour, coconut flour, walnuts, ground chia, baking powder, salt, and pumpkin pie spice in a large mixing cup. Mix once well blended with all ingredients.

3.   In a mixing cup, position the egg whites and use the electric mixer to beat until stiff peaks develop.

4.   Beat the egg yolks for about 30 seconds in the third large mixing bowl. Add honey, vanilla extract, almond milk, apple cider vinegar, and pumpkin puree. Whisk when well mixed with all ingredients.

5.   Include the dry ingredients in the egg yolk mixture and swirl to blend using a rubber spatula.

6.   Fold the whipped egg albumins carefully into the mixture, but be careful not to overmix the egg whites and deflate them.

7.   Divide the mixture uniformly into 6 wells of a muffin tin, silicone muffin cups, or silicone muffin pan.

8.   Bake for 25 - 30 minutes until the tops are gently browned, and a toothpick can be inserted in the middle and removed without sticking to it. (Start testing at the mark of 22 minutes).

FOR THE MARSHMALLOW FROSTING:

1.   Place a heatproof bowl over a saucepan filled with around 1 inch of the simmering water to set up a double boiler. Ensure the bowl shouldn't hit the water, and the pan's bottom is suspended over the waterline.

2.   Place the egg albumin, sweetener, tartar cream, and salt in a bowl and whisk for 4 minutes with the electric mixer or an electric whisk.

3.   Remove a bowl from the heat and begin whisking for 7 - 9 minutes until frosting becomes thick, or shift the mixture to the stand mixer. Gently add in the vanilla extract until the frosting is smooth and thick.

4.   Spoon the frosting back into a pipe and pipe the marshmallow frosting for each cupcake.

5.   Sprinkle a small pinch of a pumpkin pie spice with each cupcake before serving. Place the leftovers for up to 3 days in the refrigerator.

Snack Recipes

21 Jalapeno Stuffed Hamburger Steak Bites

Servings: 8 | **Time:** 25 mins | **Difficulty**: Easy

Nutrients per serving: Calories: 262 kcal | Fat: 23g | Carbohydrates: 2g | Protein: 10g | Fiber: 1g

Ingredients

For an Avocado Ranch:

2 tsp. of Worcestershire sauce

1/3 cup of avocado

1 tsp. of creole mustard

1 clove garlic

1 ½ tsp. Hot sauce

½ tsp. salt

½ Tbsp. parsley (Dried)

½ cup unsweetened almond milk

½ cup mayonnaise

¼ tsp. Onion powder

½ tsp. of Italian seasoning

For Steak Bites:

2 tsp. Worcestershire Sauce

1 tsp. salt

1 lb ground beef 80/20

1 fresh jalapeno (seeded, deveined and finely diced)

½ tsp. Garlic powder

½ tsp. Fiesta Brand Fajita Seasoning (Salt-Free)

¼ tsp. black pepper

¼ cup purple onion (finely diced)

Method

Avocado Ranch preparation:

1.   In the blender, first mix the mayo and then the next 8 ingredients and mix until smooth and blended. Whisk in the

dried herbs and pour into a cup, cover, and cool before ready to eat.

Steak Bites preparation:

1.   Cut off the ground beef in the medium mixing bowl, and then add the next seven ingredients. Mix softly, blending all the meat with the seasoning and vegetables. The meat mixture or even the steak bites would be dense. You wouldn't want to over mix or execute more. Divide the mixture into 8 pieces equally, roll each potion softly into a ball, and then flatten it to around 1⁄4 inch thick. For all 8 parts, repeat.

2.   Over medium-high heat, preheat the heavy skillet. Add up the 4 patties and cook for around 3 minutes/side or achieve the ideal point.

3.   Serve hot with the Ranch Avocado

22   Roasted Cauliflower with Chili Lime & Browned Better

Servings: 4 | **Time:** 40 mins | **Difficulty:** Easy

Nutrients per serving: Calories: 207 kcal | Fat: 18g | Carbohydrates: 9g | Protein: 3g | Fiber: 3g

Ingredients

6 Tbsp. butter melted

1/2 Tbsp. kosher salt

1/2 fresh lime

1 tsp. chili powder

1 head fresh cauliflower, dried

1 dash -1/8 tsp cayenne pepper

½ Tbsp. Granulated garlic

¼ tsp. cumin

¼ tsp paprika

Method

1. Preheat the oven to 425 °F and set aside a sheet pan with the lined-parchment.

2. Place the florets of the cauliflower in a wide cup. In a small bowl and wick, mix melted butter and the other 6 ingredients to combine. Toss the butter and spices with the florets until they are fully covered.

3. Disperse the florets on the ready sheet pan and bake for 25 to 30 minutes at 425 °F or until the florets become golden brown; whisk during the baking period. Remove from the oven and strain the florets with fresh lime. Now immediately serve.

23   Keto Chili Cheese Bites

Servings: 36 bites | **Time:** 15 mins | **Difficulty:** Easy

Nutrients per serving: Calories: 81 kcal | Fat: 6g | Carbohydrates: 0g | Protein: 3g | Fiber: 0g

Ingredients

8 oz. cream cheese, softened

6 pieces crispy cooked bacon (chopped finely)

4 cups Colby jack cheese (shredded)

1/4 tsp. salt

1/2 tsp. paprika

1 tsp. Worcestershire sauce

1 tsp. hot sauce

1 tsp. granulated garlic

1 scallion or green onion (thinly sliced)

1 1/2 tsp. chili powder (divided)

Method

1.   Mix melted cream cheese, onion, garlic, paprika, shredded cheese, 1 tsp in a large mixing cup. Chili powder, sauce from Worcestershire, sweet sauce, and salt. To blend, balance well. In a stand or portable mixer, you can mix this as well.

2.   Mix finely chopped bacon and half tsp of the chili powder in a pie plate or other flat dishes. Roll the mixture of cheese into 1″ cubes. Then roll each ball in the crumbs of bacon, pressing them into the cheese mixture gently. To smooth them out, roll each cheese ball in your palms. Refrigerate then for 1 hour.

24 Creamy Mashed Turnips

Servings: 6 | **Time:** 30 mins | **Difficulty:** Easy

Nutrients per serving: Calories: 128 kcal | Fat: 46g | Carbohydrates: 7g | Protein: 21g | Fiber: 2g

Ingredients

salt & pepper to taste

Chopped Green Onion or Chive for Garnish

5 medium turnips of baseball-sized (peeled & diced)

3 tbsp butter

2 tsp kosher salt

2 tbsp heavy cream

2 oz cream cheese

1/4 tsp Lakanto Monkfruit Sweetener

Method

1.   Add the turnips to the big pot of cold water (approximately 6 cups) and add 2 tsp of salt and sweetener to the water, if necessary. Boil and then reduce to the simmer and cook for around 20 minutes until smooth and tender.

2.   Drain the turnips well, and return to the pot. Let it hang for a minute or 2 to evaporate some of the excess moisture.

3.   Include the cream cheese, sugar, cream, and mash until you achieve the perfect consistency. To taste, season with salt and pepper. Use an immersion blender if you like a smoother consistency.

25   GG's Oil & Vinegar Coleslaw

Servings: 4-6 | **Time:** 20 mins | **Difficulty:** Easy

Nutrients per serving: Calories: 224 kcal | Fat: 46g | Carbohydrates: 7g | Protein: 21g | Fiber: 2g

Ingredients

4 T red wine vinegar

3 T finely diced purple onion

3 cups cabbage (shredded)

2 2.5 oz cans - sliced black olives (drained)

1/3 cup light olive oil or avocado oil

1 cup diced English cucumber

1 cup diced celery

1 cup diced bell pepper

1 4oz jar diced pimentos (drained)

1 ½ tsp salt

½ tsp onion powder

½ tsp dry mustard

¼ tsp Pyure (or 1 tsp of your preferred sweetener)

¼ tsp pepper

¼ tsp granulated garlic

Method

1.   In a wide dish, mix the first 7 ingredients.

2.   Whisk together the vinegar, seasonings, and the sweetener of choice in a medium dish. Slowly stir the oil into the seasonings and vinegar.

3.   Pour dressing over the vegetables with oil and vinegar and toss to coat.

4.   Cool at least an hour before serving. The longer it remains, the cooler it gets. Store it in the freezer.

26 Spicy Salmon Cucumber Bites

Servings: 4 | **Time**: 20 mins | **Difficulty:** Easy

Nutrients per serving: Calories: 112 kcal | Fat: 11g | Carbohydrates: 4g | Protein: 1g | Fiber: 1g

Ingredients

Ground black pepper

Diamond Crystal kosher salt

4 cherry tomatoes quartered

1 tbsp shallots minced

1 tbsp chives chopped

1 English cucumber (peeled and cut into ¾-inch thick slices)

1 bunch chive sprigs garnish

½ lb cooked salmon

¼ tsp Tabasco sauce

¼ tsp smoked paprika

¼ cup Paleo mayonnaise

Method

1. In a shallow dish, mix the smoked paprika, mayo, and Tabasco and blend thoroughly. If you like spicy stuff, taste the seasoning and add further Tabasco.

2. Grab the cooked flake and salmon into large bite-sized pieces.

3. Put the salmon, chives, salt, diced shallots, and pepper in a dish and mix the spicy mayonnaise gently.

4. Grab the cucumber slices, then scoop out the middle of each cucumber slice using a melon baller or tsp. Do not dig too hard, or it will turn into open-ended tubes for your cups, and the salmon filling may fall right through.

5. Divide a salmon mixture in each cup and apply a cherry tomato slice and a few chive tops.

27   Crispy Mushroom Chips

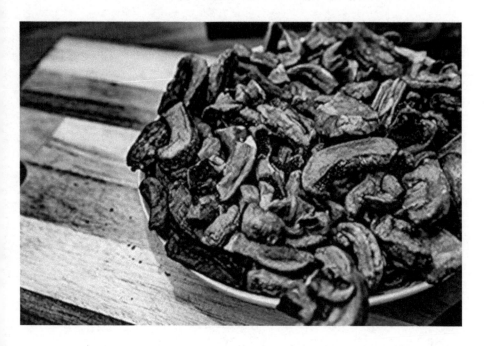

Servings: 2 | **Time:** 1 hr | **Difficulty**: Easy

Nutrients per serving: Calories: 171 kcal | Fat: 15g | Carbohydrates: 9g | Protein: 5g | Fiber: 3g

Ingredients

Kosher salt

Freshly ground pepper

2 tbsp avocado oil or melted ghee

10 oz. 300 grams of king oyster mushrooms

Method

1.   Preheat the oven to 300 °F (or 275 °F on convection baking) and use parchment paper to line several rimmed baking sheets. You'll either need to use several trays or bake in many batches for this recipe.

2.   Split the mushrooms lengthwise in half, and then cut them into 1/8-inch slices using a mandolin slicer.

3.   On the parchment-lined baking sheets, assemble the slices into a single layer. Make sure you have super-dry mushrooms and leave some room between the slices.

4.   Brush all sides of the mushroom slices with avocado oil or melted ghee, and season with pepper and salt to taste.

5.   Bake until the chips become golden brown and crispy, or for 45 minutes to an hour. If they are out of the microwave, these chips will not begin to crisp, so do not take them out if they are already sort of fluffy.

28   Chili Lime Chicken Wings

Servings: 10 | **Time:** 1 hr 45 mins | **Difficulty**: Easy

Nutrients per serving: Calories: 588 kcal | Fat: 25g | Carbohydrates: 5g | Protein: 27g | Fiber: 1g

Ingredients

Zest from 2 limes

Freshly ground pepper

6 lb chicken wings and drumsticks

4 limes cut into wedges

3 garlic cloves peeled

2 tbsp Paleo-friendly fish sauce Red Boat.

2 tbsp coconut aminos

2 jalapeno peppers or 1 serrano pepper

1-2 tbsp melted fat of choice

½ medium onion roughly chopped

½ cup cilantro tightly packed

¼ cup lime juice

Method

1.   In a blender, mix the onion, peppers, cilantro, ground pepper, garlic, lime zest & juice, fish sauce, coconut aminos, and process until the bright green purée appears.

2.   In a wide bowl, put the chicken wings and add the marinade. In your palms, blend well.

3.   Marinate the chicken for about 30 minutes and up to 12 hours in the refrigerator. For more than 12 hours, the wings should not marinate because the acid can make the beef mushy.

4.   Remove the wings from the fridge 30 minutes before you expect to roast them.

5.   These chicken wings can be baked either in the oven or on your backyard barbecue if you can stand the cold weather outside.

6.   Arrange a rack in the oven center, and on convection roast, preheat it to 400 ° F (or 425 ° F on the standard-setting). Cover with foil on a rimmed baking sheet and put a wire rack on top. Then set the wings for 30 minutes or when the wings become golden brown on the oiled wire rack and roast them.

7.   If you are grilling chicken wings, then first use the long-handled tongs with the wad of paper towels dipped in molten fat

to oil the cooking griddle. Then cook the wings on medium-hot coals for around 15 minutes, rotating once, until the fat is made and the skin becomes crisp and golden, or with the gas grill burners that set to medium.

8.   Serve with wedges of lime, and let the frenzied feeding begin.

29 Crispy Prosciutto Chips

Servings: 12 | **Time:** 20 mins | **Difficulty**: Easy

Nutrients per serving: Calories: 355 kcal | Fat: 34g | Carbohydrates: 1g | Protein: 11g

Ingredients

3 oz. of very thinly sliced Prosciutto di Parma

Method

1.   Having the rack in the center, preheat the oven to 350°F.

2.   With a piece of parchment paper, line the rimmed baking sheet, and put the prosciutto on top in a single layer. Don't overcrowd the pigs; otherwise, it won't be appropriately crisp.

3.   Place the tray in the oven until the oven is ready. Bake for about 10-15 minutes or until crunchy (based on the slices of prosciutto). To make sure they don't burn, watch those chips like a hawk.

4.   To cool, move the chips onto a wire rack. (As they cool, they get crunchier).

30   Brussels Sprouts Chips

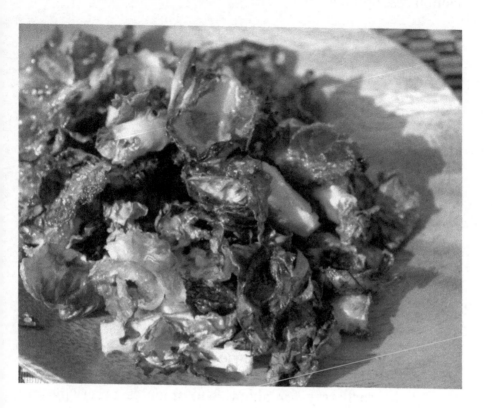

Servings: 2 | **Time:** 15 mins | **Difficulty:** Easy

Nutrients per serving: Calories: 169 kcal | Fat: 15g | Carbohydrates: 8g | Protein: 3g | Fiber: 3g

Ingredients

Lemon zest optional

Kosher salt to taste

2 tbsp melted ghee olive oil or avocado oil

2 cups Brussels sprout leaves

Method

1.   Preheat the oven to 350 °F.

2.   In a wide cup, mix the leaves, salt, and ghee (or avocado oil).

3.   Line two large parchment baking trays. Divide the leaves uniformly on each tray into a single sheet.

4.   Bake each tray for about 8-10 minutes or crispy and brown across the edges.

5.   Microplane over the chips with some lemon zest (optional), then chow immediately.

31 Green Pork and Shiitake Sliders

Servings: 6 | **Time:** 35 mins | **Difficulty:** Easy

Nutrients per serving: Calories: 346 kcal | Fat: 27g | Carbohydrates: 8g | Protein: 18g | Fiber: 4g

Ingredients

6 reconstituted shiitake mushrooms (dried & finely chopped)

2 large eggs lightly beaten

1/8 cup coconut flour up to 1/4 cup

1/4 cup full-fat coconut milk

1/2 cup yellow onion (finely chopped)

1/2 cup fresh cilantro leaves

1/2 cup celery small-diced (around 2 medium stalks)

1 tbsp Red Boat fish sauce

1 tbsp coconut oil (or fat of choice)

1 tbsp coconut aminos

1 lb ground pork

1 lb frozen chopped spinach

1.5 tsp freshly ground black pepper

1 tsp Diamond Crystal kosher salt

Method

1.   In a secure microwave dish, pour the frozen spinach and cover it with a lid. To defrost it, microwave the bowl on top for about 4 minutes.

2.   In a colander, put the defrosted spinach and press all the liquid out.

3.   In a large cast-iron skillet, heat 1 tbsp coconut oil over medium heat.

4.   Toss along with salt & pepper to taste in the onions (chopped) and mushrooms. Sauté the ingredients unless they've evaporated the liquid and softened the onions.

5.   Use a hand blender, blitz the coconut milk, cilantro, and celery.

6.   Replace the spinach, puree, mushrooms, onions, eggs, coconut flour (1/8 cup), coconut aminos, fish sauce, pepper, and salt, and put the ground pork in a big dish.

7.   Mix all the ingredients gently

8.   Shape into the tiny patties of the meat mixture (2 inches in diameter).

9.   Heat 2 tsp of coconut oil on medium heat in a cast-iron skillet (the oil should make a thin layer). Fry the sliders on both sides for 3 minutes.

32 Broiled Herb-Stuffed Sardines

Servings: 3 | **Time:** 25 mins | **Difficulty:** Easy

Nutrients per serving: Calories: 415 kcal | Fat: 36g | Carbohydrates: 5g | Protein: 20g | Fiber: 2g

Ingredients

1 large lemon

1/2 cup Italian parsley (chopped)

2 tbsp oil

3 tbsp butter or ghee

4 green onion stalks (chopped)

6 large fresh sardines

2 lb Diamond Crystal kosher salt

Freshly ground black pepper

Method

1. Preheat the broiler to a high degree and put the top rack four inches from the heating unit.

2. Take the kitchen knife out of it and gut the fish. Cut out a shallow path around the fish's belly and take the innards out. Rinse the fish, then pat it dry.

3. In the food processor, put along the butter or ghee, green onions, salt, parsley, and pepper. Pulse until you have formed a uniform paste.

4. Spoon each sardine cavity with 1 tbsp of filling.

5. Brush the fish's skin with the molten bacon fat and sprinkle on top with salt and pepper.

6. Place the ready-made sardines on top of the foil-lined baking sheet on a wire rack and place them in the oven.

7. Broil for about 5 minutes, tossing at the halfway point with the cod.

8. Spritz the new lemon juice with it.

33 Oven-Roasted Tomatoes

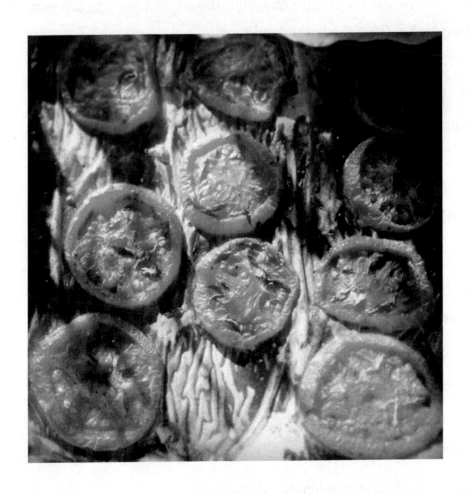

Servings: 2 | **Time:** 55 mins | **Difficulty:** Easy

Nutrients per serving: Calories: 185 kcal | Fat: 15g | Carbohydrates: 13g | Protein: 3g | Fiber: 4g

Ingredients

1 tbsp Sunny Paris seasoning (or your preferred dried herb blend)

10 plum tomatoes (Choose a tomato type with more flesh & fewer seeds).

2 tbsp extra virgin olive oil (or your favorite fat)

Diamond Crystal kosher salt

Freshly ground black pepper

Method

1.   Preheat the 400 F toaster oven and sweep up the tomatoes.

2.   Slice the tomatoes in half lengthwise and scatter them on a single sheet on the foil-lined baking tray, in a cut-side-up position.

3.   Sprinkle the seasoning mixture of dried spices, salt, and pepper on tomatoes and the virgin olive oil (extra).

4.   Pop the tray in an oven and roast these tomatoes for about 45 minutes, turning the tray several times to cook uniformly. Tomatoes are finished when the sides are a little brown, shrunk a little, and soft and chewy.

34   Simple Crab Salad

Servings: 4 | **Time**: 10 mins | **Difficulty**: Easy

Nutrients per serving: Calories: 146 kcal | Fat: 6g | Carbohydrates: 1g | Protein: 21g | Fiber: 1g

Ingredients

1 lb cooked lump crab meat

1 tbsp lemon juice

2 scallions thinly sliced

2 tbsp chopped Italian parsley

2 tbsp paleo mayonnaise

Diamond Crystal kosher salt

Freshly ground black pepper

Method

1.   Assemble and cut your herbs with your ingredients. Crack open the 'o crab can' and squeeze the excess liquid out.

2.   In a medium-sized dish, pour the crab and blend in the scallions, salt, parsley, and pepper.

3.   Next, in a separate bowl, put the mayonnaise and lemon juice together. When mixed, apply the combination of mayonnaise to the crab dish. Taste it to see if more mayo, salt, lemon juice, or pepper is required.

4.   Serve it with avocado or guacamole over the greens. Or, if you're looking to put a short appetizer together, mix the crab salad with several finely diced red bell pepper, then spoon it into some spears of endive.

35 Green Sliders

Servings: 6 | **Time:** 50 mins | **Difficulty:** Easy

Nutrients per serving: Calories: 354 kcal | Fat: 27g | Carbohydrates: 10g | Protein: 20g | Fiber: 5g

Ingredients

1 medium garlic clove (minced)

1 lb frozen spinach (chopped)

1 lb ground beef

1 tbsp unsalted butter (or coconut oil)

1 tsp Diamond Crystal kosher salt

1.5 tsp freshly ground black pepper

1/2 cup celery (small-dice)

1/2 cup Italian parsley leaves loosely packed

1/2 cup medium yellow onion (chopped)

1/2 lb cremini mushrooms (finely chopped)

1/4 cup coconut cream (or coconut milk)

1/4 cup coconut flour

1/4 tsp freshly grated nutmeg

2 large eggs beaten

2 tbsp coconut oil for frying Fleur de sel

Method

1.   Pour the spinach box into a microwaveable bowl and then microwave it on high to defrost it for about 4 minutes. (Without an oven, you should even let it defrost overnight).

2.   In a colander, put the defrosted spinach and press all the liquid out.

3.   In the large cast-iron skillet, heat the butter or the coconut oil on medium heat and toss in chopped onions & mushrooms with salt & pepper.

4.   Sauté the vegetables until they have evaporated the liquid and softened the onions. In a wide dish, add the ground beef. Just put aside.

5.   Put in a dish of coconut milk, celery and parsley and mix with a hand blender.

6.   Pour it on the ground beef until a puree is developed, and then include the chopped spinach, garlic, measured salt &

pepper, coconut flour, fresh nutmeg, beaten eggs, and a mixture of cooked mushrooms.

7.　　Mix all the ingredients gently and shape little patties with the meat mixture (about 2 inches in diameter). There are about 30 patties you can have.

8.　　In a cast-iron skillet, heat 2 tbsp of coconut oil on medium heat and cook the sliders in 3 batches. Cook the sliders on either side for 3 minutes.

9.　　Place the patties on the plate until they're finished cooking. Dig in for a heated sauce of marinara

36   Roasted Portobello Mushrooms

Servings: 4 | **Time:** 35 mins | **Difficulty:** Easy

Nutrients per serving: Calories: 51 kcal | Fat: 4g | Carbohydrates: 3g | Protein: 2g | Fiber: 1g

Ingredients

Sunny Paris seasoning (or your preferred salt-free herb blend) Minced fresh herbs optional

Melted ghee melted coconut oil (or your preferred fat)

Lemon or lime juice (or your preferred vinegar)

Kosher salt

Freshly ground pepper

4 large Portobello mushrooms (clean with a paper towel or damp cloth)

Method

1.   Preheat oven to 400 °F. Put an aluminum foil on the middle rack or a parchment-lined baking dish.

2.   Grab and cut the stems from the mushrooms, scrape the gills with a spoon, and turn down the gill- side caps.

3.   On top of each mushroom, cut a shallow 'X,' brush the entire cap (top & bottom) with molten fat, and season with salt and pepper on both sides.

4.   Before sticking these on a hot baking tray in an oven, sprinkle a few Sunny Paris seasoning (or your preferred salt-free herb blend) over the caps, gill-side up.

5.   For 10 minutes, roast the shrooms and then flip them to cook for an extra 10 minutes (total 20 minutes). If the cooking caps are used as buns, you are done.

6.   Cut them up and then squeeze some lemon juice and the minced fresh herbs if you are eating the shrooms as a side dish.

37 Cauliflower and Carrot Puree

Servings: 6 | **Time:** 40 mins | **Difficulty:** Easy

Nutrients per serving: Calories: 138 kcal | Fat: 11g | Carbohydrates: 9g | Protein: 2g | Fiber: 3g

Ingredients

Splash of heavy cream optional

Freshly ground black pepper

Diamond Crystal kosher salt

4 tbsp ghee (or fat of choice)

3 large carrots (cut into small chunks)

2 garlic cloves (minced)

1 large cauliflower cut up into florets

½ medium onion coarsely (chopped)

¼ cup of water

¼ cup organic chicken broth

Method

1.   Chop up your vegetables and, over medium heat, melt 3 tbsp of ghee in a big stockpot.

2.   Within the bubbling fat, put the veggies, broth, and water. Cover the pot as the liquid begins to boil, turn the heat down to the minimum, and let it steam until softened (25-30 minutes). Make sure don't dry your pot.

3.   Add another tbsp of ghee, the splashes of heavy cream, salt, and pepper, and mix until creamy, using an immersion mixer.

38 Sausage and Spinach Stuffed Portobello Mushrooms

Servings: 5 | **Time:** 1 hr 5 mins | **Difficulty**: Easy

Nutrients per serving: Calories: 425 kcal | Fat: 35g | Carbohydrates: 11g | Protein: 20g | Fiber: 4g

Ingredients

Sunny Paris seasoning

Freshly ground black pepper

Diamond Crystal kosher salt

avocado oil (or cooking fat of choice)

5 medium portobello mushrooms

2 tbsp ghee (or fat of choice)

1½ cups marinara sauce

1 tbsp coconut flour

1 lb uncooked sausage (removed from its casing)

1 large egg lightly beaten

½ small onion minced

½ lb frozen spinach (defrosted & squeezed dried)

Method

1.   Keep the rack in the middle of the oven, preheat an oven to 400° F, and put the foil-lined baking sheet over the rack.

2.   Gather your shrooms, wipe the tops with a moist cloth, and take a spoon from the stems and gills. Place them in the shallow baking dish until washed.

3.   Using a sharp paring knife, cut a shallow "X" on the top of each shroom and brush an avocado oil in the shrooms, and salt and pepper season the tops & bottoms.

4.   Place the mushrooms in the oven, position the gill side up, and then bake for 10 minutes on a pre- heated baking sheet. Flip each mushroom and cook them down on the gill side for an extra 10 minutes. Take the tray from the oven and leave to cool at room temperature for the mushrooms.

5.   To broil, raise the oven temperature.

6.   You should start preparing the stuffing when the mushrooms are cooking. Heat the ghee over medium heat in a large skillet and sauté the diced onion (with salt & pepper) until tender and translucent.

7.   Apply to the pan the bacon and a few dashes of a Sunny Paris seasoning. Cook the meat until the meat is not pink anymore.

8.   Remove a meat mixture and leave it to cool at room temperature in a medium cup.

9.   Add the egg, coconut flour, spinach, salt, and pepper until the sausage is cooled and blended. Shift now this cooled roasted mushrooms to another foil-lined baking sheet (lots of mushroom liquid would be on the initial baking sheet), layer the stuffing on each shell, and press down to make it more compact.

10.   For around 5 minutes, put the tray under a broiler (center rack), rotating halfway during the cooking process.

11.   When the mushrooms are full, the stuffing should be uniformly browned (not burned).

12.   Add marinara sauce to the stuffed mushrooms and serve instantly.

39 Roasted Portobello Mushroom Packets with Garlic, Shallots, and Balsamic Vinegar

Servings: 5 | **Time:** 40 mins | **Difficulty:** Easy

Nutrients per serving: Calories: 141 kcal | Fat: 12g | Carbohydrates: 7g | Protein: 2g | Fiber: 2g

Ingredients

1 tbsp Balsamic vinegar

10-15 garlic cloves peeled

2 medium shallots (coarsely chopped)

3 tbsp ghee or fat of choice

5 large Portobello mushrooms tops (wiped clean, stems & gills removed)

Diamond Crystal kosher salt

extra virgin olive oil

Freshly ground black pepper

Method

1.   Preheat an oven to 400°F and cut the shallots coarsely, and trim the garlic ends. In a food processor, throw the shallots to finely mince them (or mince by hand).

2.   In a 3:1 fat to vinegar ratio, apply fat and vinegar to the minced alliums. By using an acceptable salt and fresh ground black pepper sprinkling, season this vinaigrette mixture.

3.   Place each of the Portobello mushrooms, stem side up, on a sheet of heavy-duty aluminum foil. Each shroom is lightly coated with some extra virgin olive oil and salt and pepper. Put into each mushroom a dollop of vinaigrette, spreading unless the cap is filled.

4.   Seal every mushroom packet tightly and put it on a baking tray. In the microwave, stick the tray and roast for about 25 minutes.

5.   Take the mushrooms from the packages and slice them up.

40 Collard Greens

Servings: 4 | **Time:** 30 mins | **Difficulty**: Easy

Nutrients per serving: Calories: 138 kcal | Fat: 9g | Carbohydrates: 14g | Protein: 12g | Fiber: 9g

Ingredients

Freshly squeezed lemon juice (or balsamic vinegar)

Freshly cracked black pepper

3 cloves of garlic minced

2 lb assertive greens (such as collards, kale, mustard, or turnip greens; coarsely chopped and stemmed)

1½ tsp Diamond Crystal brand kosher salt

1 tbsp olive oil

1 cup diced ham (or bacon optional)

¼ cup chicken broth

Method

1.   In a deep kettle, boil 2 quarts of water. Include the greens and salt and whisk until wilted. Cover it and cook until just tender (approx 7 minutes) for the greens.

2.   In a colander, rinse the collard greens. To cool the pot, clean it with cold water and refill it with cold water and a few ice cubes. To pause the cooking process, pour the greens into the ice water.

3.   Shift the greens back to a colander and put a small handful to squeeze out much water as possible into a potato ricer. Repeat unless all the greens are no soggier any more. In a locked jar in the freezer, you can store these greens for up to 4 days.

4.   Now you're set for the greens to sauté. If you need your greens to be sliced smaller, do it now.

5.   Over medium heat, heat a big skillet. When the pan is warmed, stir in the olive oil.

6.   Then throw in some bacon or ham and add your fried collard greens. Top with 1/4 cup of chicken broth and cover for 2 minutes. When required, taste and change with salt & pepper, and squeeze a lemon juice or vinegar.

Beverages Recipes

41 Low Carb German Gingerbread Hot Chocolate

Servings: 2 | **Time**: 20 mins | **Difficulty**: Easy

Nutrients per serving: Calories: 72 kcal | Fat: 4g | Carbohydrates: 11g | Protein: 3g | Fiber: 5g

Ingredients

1/4 Cup Cocoa Powder, Unsweetened

2 Cups Chocolate Almond Milk, Unsweetened

1/2 Tsp. Liquid Stevia

1/4 Cup Stevia

1/4 Tsp. Cardamom, Ground

1 Tsp. Cinnamon, Ground

1/8 Tsp. Allspice, Ground

1/8 Tsp. Anise Seed, Ground

1/8 Tsp. Cloves, Ground

1/8 Tsp. Nutmeg, Ground

1/8 Tsp. Ginger, Ground

Method

1.   Combine all the ingredients in a saucepan and heat it over medium heat.

2.   Once it boils, reduce the heat to low, and let it simmer for about 5 minutes with intermittent stirring.

3.   Decant into serving mugs and enjoy.

42   Coconut Pumpkin Steamer

Servings: 1 | **Time:** 5 mins | **Difficulty:** Easy

Nutrients per serving: Calories: 241 kcal | Fat: 24g | Carbohydrates: 9g | Protein: 2g | Fiber: 1g

Ingredients

1 Tsp. Vanilla Extract

1/2 Cup Coconut Milk

Stevia, To Taste

1/4 Tsp. Pumpkin Pie Spice, Without Sugar

Method

1.   Combine all the ingredients in a saucepan and heat it over medium heat.

2.   Once the bubbles start to form, take off the heat, and serve warm.

43 Low Carb Margarita Mix

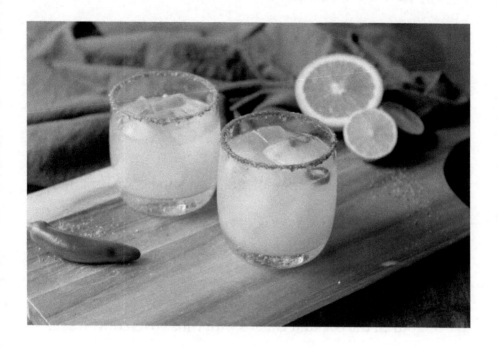

Servings: 2 | **Time:** 5 mins | **Difficulty:** Easy

Nutrients per serving: Calories: 35 kcal | Fat: 0g | Carbohydrates: 9g | Protein: 0g | Fiber: 0g

Ingredients

1/2 Cup Lemon Juice, Fresh

1 & 1/2 Cups Water

1/4 Tsp. Liquid Stevia

1/3 Cup Erythritol, Powdered

1/8 Tsp. Orange Extract

1 Cup Tequila Ice, To Taste

Method

1.   Combine all the ingredients in a pitcher except tequila and ice.

2.   Mix well to dissolve the sweetener.

3.   Add the tequila and stir.

4.   Pour in the cocktail glasses with rims covered with salt.

5.   Add the ice and enjoy.

44 Low Carb Electrolyte Water

Servings: 4 | **Time:** 5 mins | **Difficulty**: Easy

Nutrients per serving: Calories: 2 kcal | Fat: 0g | Carbohydrates: 1g | Protein: 0g

Ingredients

4 Cups Water

2 Tbsps. Lemon Juice

1/8 Tsp. Baking Soda

Stevia, To Taste

1/8 Tsp. Salt

Method

1.   Combine all the ingredients in a bottle, cover it, and shake well.

2.   Serve and enjoy.

45 Low Carb Pumpkin Spice Mocha

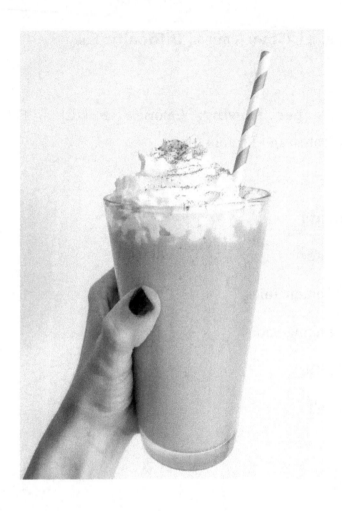

Servings: 2 | **Time:** 15 mins | **Difficulty**: Easy

Nutrients per serving: Calories: 187 kcal | Fat: 21g | Carbohydrates: 1g | Protein: 0g

Ingredients

1 Tsp. Pumpkin Pie Spice, Without Sugar

Stevia, To Taste

3 Tbsps. Cocoa Butter

1/4 Cup Coffee Grounds

3 Cups Water

Method

1.   Brew the coffee according to your preference with the pumpkin spice in it.

2.   Add the cocoa butter in it and blend with an immersion blender until a smooth consistency is attained and it becomes frothy.

3.   Add the desired quantity of sweetener and enjoy.

46 Kombucha Sangria

Servings: 7 | **Time:** 10 mins | **Difficulty:** Easy

Nutrients per serving: Calories: 101 kcal | Fat: 0g | Carbohydrates: 6.5g | Protein: 0.1g | Fiber: 0g

Ingredients

4 Tbsps. Monkfruit, Powdered

1 Cup Orange Juice

2 Cups Kombucha

3 & 1/4 Cups Spanish Wine

1 Lime, Sliced

1 Orange, Sliced

1 Lemon, Sliced

1/2 Cup Brandy (Optional)

Method

1.   Combine all the ingredients in a pitcher, except orange, lemon, and lime slices.

2.   Stir well to mix and add the orange, lemon, and lime slices.

3.   Serve with ice and enjoy.

47 Pumpkin Spice Hot Buttered Rum

Servings: 4 | **Time**: 10 mins | **Difficulty**: Easy

Nutrients per serving: Calories: 73 kcal | Fat: 60g | Carbohydrates: 1.2g | Protein: 0.2g | Fiber: 0.5g

Ingredients

1 Cup Butter

1 Cup Golden Monkfruit

3 Tbsps. Maple Syrup, Sugar-Free

2 Tsps. Vanilla Extract

1 Cup Heavy Cream

1 & 1/2 Cups Monkfruit, Powdered

1 Tbsp. Pumpkin Pie Spice

2 Cups Hot Water

1 Cup Rum

Method

1.   Take a bowl and put the golden Monkfruit, butter, vanilla, and maple syrup in it. Whisk well for few minutes until creamy and fluffy.

2.   Add all the other ingredients except rum and water and mix well. Set aside.

3.   Fill each serving glass with 1/4 cup Rum, 1/2 cup water, and two to three tbsps. of the batter and stir well.

48 Tart Cherry Lemon Drop

Servings: 1 | **Time:** 5 mins | **Difficulty:** Easy

Nutrients per serving: Calories: 660 kcal | Fat: 60g | Carbohydrates: 7g | Protein: 13g | Fiber: 7g

Ingredients

4 Tbsps. Tart Cherry Juice

4 Lemon Wedges

2 Tbsps. Fresh Lemon Juice

3 Tbsps. Vodka

2 Tbsps. Water

1 Tbsp. Monkfruit, Powdered

1 Tbsp. Lemon Juice, Fresh

1 Tsp. Monkfruit, Granular

Ice, To Taste

Method

1.   Combine powdered lemon juice, water, and lemon wedges in a blender and blend well until a smooth consistency is attained.

2.   Add the vodka, tart cherry juice, and ice in it and blend again until desires consistency.

3.   Dip the rim of the cocktail glass in lemon juice and then in granular Monkfruit.

4.   Pour in the juice and garnish with a lemon slice if you want.

49   Orange Creamsicle Mimosas

Servings: 1 | **Time**: 10 mins | **Difficulty:** Easy

Nutrients per serving: Calories: 255 kcal | Fat: 11.5g | Carbohydrates: 8g | Protein: 0.9g | Fiber: 0.1g

Ingredients

1 Tbsp. Vanilla Vodka

1/4 Cup Orange Juice, Fresh

2 Tbsps. Heavy Cream

1 Tsp. Monkfruit, Powdered

1/2 Cup Sparkling Wine, Dry (Prosecco Or Champagne)

Method

1.   Combine all the ingredients in a blender except wine. Blend it well until a smooth consistency is attained.

2.   Add the wine and serve.

50 Low Carb Strawberry Basil Bourbon Smash

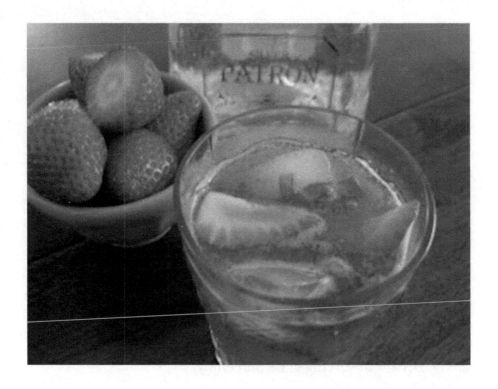

Servings: 1 | **Time:** 10 mins | **Difficulty**: Easy

Nutrients per serving: Calories: 159 kcal | Fat: 0.4g | Carbohydrates: 3.5g | Protein: 0.5g | Fiber: 0.9g

Ingredients

1/4 Cup Bourbon

3 Basil Leaves

1/8 Tsp. Black Pepper, Ground

3 Strawberries, Sliced

2 Tbsps. Lemon Juice, Fresh

1 Tsp. Erythritol, Powdered

Ice, To Taste

Method

1.   Combine all the ingredients in a blender and blend until desired consistency is attained.

2.   Decant in serving glass and enjoy.

Lightning Source UK Ltd.
Milton Keynes UK
UKHW022031060521
383282UK00003B/328